# The Bone Broth Secret

## The Ultimate Culinary Adventure Health, Beauty, Longevity and Weight Loss (30 Delicious Broth & Soup Recipes to Improve Your Health, Inflammation, Lose Weight and Reverse Aging, Bone Broth Diet, Lose Weight Fast)

By:

**Melvin Schmitt**

Published by Shepal Publishing

# Table of Contents

# Introduction

Bone broths and stocks have been around for millennia. However, it is only over the last few years that we have seen them become such a popular part of today's health conscious culinary circles. However, as much as people know about bone broth, there are many who do not know what exactly it is. Is it a soup, an ingredient, a condiment?

Bone Broth is all of those things and more. It is among the most versatile, nutritious ingredients you can have in your kitchen. Its health benefits are so profound that the LA Lakers diet has been overhauled so that it can incorporate bone broths.

Adding bone broth to your diet does not have to disrupt your eating habits, and you will soon find that it adds a pleasant dynamic to your meals. The health benefits are a bonus, and are another reason why you should add broths to your diet. This book will explore some of the benefits of bone broths, and supply you with 30 mouth-watering recipes to help you utilize bone broth every day.

# Chapter 1:
# The Benefits of Bone Broth

With its new growing popularity, the benefits of bone broths are slowly coming to light, and more people are learning how they can benefit from integrating bone broths into their diets.

For instance, bone broths contain minerals that are important to the body such as calcium, magnesium and phosphorus. These minerals are essential for functions such as healthy bone formation, and have been found to be important in reducing the development and symptoms of diseases such as arthritis.

Gelatin released from bones has also been shown to have numerous benefits. Not only is it a good source of protein, it also is important in preventing degenerative joint diseases and in strengthening tissues like ligaments and tendons.

Bone broth helps to boost the immune system by supplying the body with "non-essential" or "conditional" amino acids. These amino acids help to promote wound healing, inhibit the deterioration of muscle tissues, and can even help in the production of muscle tissue and liver cells.

The gelatin in bone broth is said to promote the production of keratin, which is vital for healthy hair, skin and nails. Many of the people who have been using bone broths for extended periods state that it has helped them keep their youthful looks.

Bone broths help to heal the gut, therefore, it should come as no surprise that they help to prevent weight gain. This is because a healthy gut is able to absorb nutrients better. In addition, the some of the minerals that are found in bone broths help to control blood sugar levels, making them the ideal supplement for people who suffer from diabetes and other sugar related illnesses.

However, one of the biggest benefits of bone broth is that it can be extremely filling. Bone broth soups and drinks are known to make you feel full for hours, while providing you with a minimal number of calories. For instance, a cup of bone broth can contain up to 14 grams of protein, yet contain the same number of calories. This is not very special, as many dietary supplements that we use today can claim the same numbers. However, bone broths are the only supplements that can claim to lack hidden sugars. Unless they are being used as an ingredient in a larger meal, bone broths will rarely contain hidden sugars from fruit and other high carbohydrate foods.

Bone broth is not only good for your health, it helps in a variety of different ways as well. It is easy on your pocket, as finding bones to make a broth is as easy as having a chicken. Bone broths also help improve people's temperament, as they can have a calming effect on the body.

You can reap these benefits by integrating a well-made bone broth into your diet. In the following chapters, you shall find some easy recipes that will help you do that with ease, and will help you wield this secret culinary weapon properly.

# Chapter 2:
# Bone Broths and Bone Broth Beverages

Bone broths are easy to make, and have been used by everyone from paupers to royalty. This chapter looks at some basic bone broth recipes and resultant beverages that you may want to try with your next meal.

## 1. Beef Bone Broth

Beef bone broth serves as one of the main ingredients for many dishes around the world, and this mouth-watering recipe is sure to be a hit among friends and family.

**Ingredients:**

- 6 lbs beef bones

- 1 lb chopped carrots

- 2 chopped onions

- 1 leek, chopped

- 6-8 liters of water

- 2 Tablespoons apple cider or white wine vinegar

- 6 sprigs fresh thyme

- 2 fresh bay leaves

## Preparation Method

- Roast the bones in an oven at 400° F for 35-40 minutes and the vegetables for 15 minutes

- Place the bones in a slow cooker, and add the water and vinegar. Simmer and set it for 24 hours

- Skim the scum off the top of the mixture as it cooks

- With about 5 hours remaining, add the roasted vegetables and herbs

- Strain the mixture when it is done, the finer the strainer the better

- Serve the broth immediately, or store it to consume later. Consume it in a week if you are refrigerating it or a year if you are freezing.

## 2. Turkey Bone Broth

This is a fantastic recipe, especially after thanksgiving. It can also be used to make Chicken Bone Broth, just substitute the turkey for two medium sized chickens

### Ingredients

- 1 trimmed turkey

- Salt

- 6-8 liters of water

- 2 roughly cut onions

- 1 roughly cut carrot

- 1 chopped celery stalk

- 2 bay leaves

- 1 teaspoon black peppercorns

- 4 sprigs thyme

- 4 sprigs rosemary

- 2 tablespoons apple cider or white wine vinegar

### Preparation Method

- Cut the turkey into pieces, lightly coat them in salt and roast in the oven at 375° F for 40 minutes

- Place the bones in a slow cooker and simmer for 8 hours

- Add vinegar and peppercorns and herbs after 1 hour

- Add vegetables with 5 hours remaining

- Pour resultant mixture through a strainer and store for later use, or consume immediately

# 3. Veal Bone Broth

Veal has a very delicate flavor. This recipe is designed to complement that flavor and provide you with a more exotic experience.

## Ingredients

- 5 lbs Veal bones

- ¾ liter red cooking wine

- ¼ cup parsley

- ¼ cup dill

- 5 roughly chopped carrots

- 4 roughly chopped celery sticks

- 2 cubed parsnips

- 2 cubed sweet potatoes

- 1 roughly chopped turnip

- Two onions cut in half.

## Preparation Method

- Roast veal bones at 450°F for 30 to 40 minutes

- Place red wine, onions, carrots, celery, parsley and dill in a pot and simmer for 15 minutes

- Place the bones and red wine mixture in a slow cooker and simmer for 22 hours

- Add remaining vegetables to the broth with 5 hours to go

- Strain the broth and consume immediately, or store for future use.

# 4. Shrimp Stock

Tires of having the same boring seafood dishes? Try this recipe as a base next time.

## Ingredients

- 2 lbs shrimp, shells only

- 2 carrots, diced

- 1 diced onion

- 1 celery stalk, diced

- A bay leaf

- A teaspoon of salt

- ¼ cup vermouth

- A teaspoon of olive oil

## Preparation Method

- Put the shrimp shells, carrots, onions, oil, bay leaf, celery and salt in a pot and cook on medium heat for 10 minutes

- Add the sherry and simmer until almost all the liquid is gone

- Cover the mixture with water and simmer for 45 minutes

- Strain the stock and allow it to cool.

- Consume immediately or store for later use

# 5. Pork Bone Broth

Pork bones are easier to find than any other bones, and the broth made from them serves as a good starting point for sauces.

## Ingredients

- 5-6 lbs Pork bones

- 5 liters of water

- 2 tablespoons white vinegar

- 2 roughly cut onions

- 1 roughly cut carrot

- 1 diced celery stalk

- 2 bay leaves

- Black peppercorns to taste

- 4 sprigs fresh thyme

## Preparation Instructions

- Roast the bones in an oven at 400°F for 40 minutes

- Place the bones in a slow cooker, add water and simmer for 15 to 20 hours

- Add the remaining ingredients after 1 hour

- Strain the broth and allow it to cool. Use immediately or store to consume later

# 6. Clove and Tomato Sipping Broth

This very simple recipe is necessary for those who are looking for a new take on tomato soups.

## Ingredients

- 12 cherry tomatoes, cut in half

- 1 tablespoon tomato puree

- 1 tablespoon butter or lard

- 3 cloves

- 2 tablespoons salt

- 1 pint Beef Bone Broth

## Preparation Instructions

- Place tomatoes, tomato puree, lard, cloves and salt in a pan and cook on low heat for 5 minutes, stirring occasionally

- Add bone broth and simmer for 5 minutes

- Using a food processor, blend the mixture and strain it. Use immediately or store for later use.

# 7. Spicy Ginger Sipping Broth

This delicate broth will prove to be an instant hit, especially among those who like a little spice with their food.

## Ingredients

- 1.5 pints Beef Bone Broth

- 2 Deseeded Serrano Chilies

- 1 small piece ginger

- 1 tablespoon butter or lard

- ¼ teaspoon powdered turmeric

- 3 teaspoons honey

- 2/3 tablespoon salt

## Preparation Instructions

- Place chilies, ginger, lard, honey, salt and turmeric in a saucepan and cook for five minutes, stirring occasionally

- Add bone broth and simmer for 10 minutes

- Use a food processor to blend the resulting liquid

- Strain it and consume immediately or store it for later use.

# 8. Bourbon Broth

This is a Bloody Mary where the Bone Broth substitutes the Tomato juice. This recipe also swaps the vodka for Bourbon, giving it a more interesting flavor.

## Ingredients

- 0.5 pint beef bone broth

- 1 shot bourbon

- ½ teaspoon Tabasco Sauce

- 3 teaspoons Tomato Juice

- 1 teaspoon Worcestershire Sauce

- Pinch of salt

- A splash of Fresh lemon juice

## Preparation Method

- Place all ingredients in a blender and mix thoroughly

- To serve hot, heat in a small pot over medium heat for 5 minutes

- Serve immediately

# 9. Spinach and Turmeric Shake

This exotic shake is healthy and nutritious, and good for breakfast or as a snack during the day.

## Ingredients

- 2 cups spinach

- 1 pint beef bone broth

- ¼ teaspoon turmeric

- 4 fl oz. apple juice

- 1 chopped apple

- 1 cup ice

- Juice from a lemon

## Preparation Instructions

- Mix the ingredients together in a food processor until smooth

- Serve immediately or store for up to 1 day

# 10. Lime and Coconut Sipping Broth

Coconut milk is very healthy, and when combined with bone broth can taste divine.

## Ingredients

- 1 pint turkey bone broth

- 4 tablespoons fresh ground ginger

- 8 fl oz. coconut milk

- Juice from two limes

- 1 teaspoon salt

## Preparation Method

- Heat all the ingredients in a small pot for 5 minutes using medium heat

- Mix together in a food processor until smooth

- Strain the resultant broth and leave to cool

- Serve immediately or store for up to a year in the freezer

## 11. Fish Bone Broth

Many people do not realise  just how rich and nutritious a good Fish bone broth can be. This recipe is sure to open your eyes to a whole new world of possibilities.

### Ingredients

- 2 average sized, whole, non-oily fish (such as Haddock or Red snapper) OR Fish bones or a cleaned fish carcass (for additional benefits, ensure you add some fish heads)

- ¼ cup apple cider vinegar

- Assorted vegetables (Adding starchy vegetables such as potatoes, parsnips, winter squash, and yams is discouraged)

- 1-2 standard yellow onions

- 2-4 carrots

- 2 bay leaves, the fresher the better

- 3 sprigs of rosemary, sage and thyme (if you cannot get fresh herbs then take 1-2 teaspoons of each herb and a bay leaf and wrap them in a cheesecloth to create a "tea bag")

- 3 sprigs parsley

- 2/3 tablespoon sea salt

## Optional additions for variety:

- 2-3 cloves garlic

- ½ inch fresh ginger

- Lemon rind from 1 lemon

- 2-3 celery stalks

## Preparation Instructions

- Wash the fish thoroughly.

- De-bone the fish, storing the meat for later use

- Place the bones, fins, tails, skins and heads into a pot

- Add the remaining ingredients and fill the pot with 1 gallon of water (or enough to cover the ingredients)

- Let the ingredients in the pot sit for at least an hour to allow the vinegar to extract the minerals from the bones

- Bring the contents of the pot to the boil, then turn the heat down and simmer for at least 4 hours

## 12. Rocket Broth

Rocket Broth is the bone broth version of the now popular "Bulletproof Coffee" and will prove just as refreshing and nourishing as its more famous cousin. In this recipe, coconut oil is used rather than MCT oil because MCT oil is usually processed (refined) coconut oil. As you probably already know, processed foods tend to lose certain beneficial properties, therefore using natural Coconut oil is more healthy.

### Ingredients

- 2 cups bone broth (Any of the Bone broth recipes in this book will do)

- Salt to taste

- 3 teaspoons ghee or butter

- 3 teaspoons coconut oil

### Preparation Method

- Warm the broth on the cooker or in the microwave for a few minutes

- Mix the warmed broth, salt, butter or ghee and coconut oil in a blender. (Removing the piece at the top of the blender and covering the hole with a tea towel will allow the warm air to escape from the blender without blowing the top of the appliance)

- Blend on max power for 1-2 minutes or until the blend is frothy and emulsified

- Pour into a cup or mug and enjoy!

If you would like to add an extra kick to the rocket broth you may add a few (3-6) teaspoons of gelatin or collagen peptides (if you did not use a gelatin rich bone broth) AFTER you have blended the broth.

# 13. Fragrant Rosemary Sipping Broth

This is one of the tastiest sipping broths you will find, and the rosemary and garlic interact perfectly to give you one of the best seasonings you have ever had to a bone broth.

## Ingredients

- 3 teaspoons olive oil

- 6 teaspoons rosemary (Fresh rosemary is recommended but you could use dried rosemary if you do not have access to any)

- 1 teaspoon salt

- Lemon juice (from at least 1 lemon)

- 1/3 tablespoon Garlic powder

- 3 cloves garlic, diced

- 3 cups of Chicken or Turkey Bone Broth

## Preparation Instructions

- Mix the oil, diced garlic and salt in a pan and cook on medium-high heat for at least 5 minutes, stirring periodically

- Add the rosemary and stir for another 2 minutes

- Introduce the lemon juice, garlic powder and bone broth to the saucepan, stirring as you do so

- Turn down the heat to about medium and let the mixture simmer for 10 – 15 minutes

- Pour the mixture into a blender and mix for at least two minutes

- Pour the result through a strainer and serve immediately in your favorite mug or pitcher.

# Chapter 3:
# Bone Broth Soups and Stews

Soups and stews made with bone broths as a base are extremely rich and flavorful, and have been known to help improve people's moods. This chapter looks at 10 recipes that are sure to become family favorites.

## 1. Continental Onion Soup

This European style Onion soup has ancient roots, and this unique take on it is an amazing way to reinvent a classic.

**Ingredients**

- 3 Tablespoons butter or lard

- 2 sliced onions

- 1 bay leaf

- 2 sprigs thyme

- 2 garlic cloves

- 1/3 tablespoon salt

- 4 fl oz. sherry

- 8 fl oz. red wine

- ½ teaspoon black pepper

- 3 pints beef bone broth

## Preparation Method

- Sauté the onions, thyme, bay leaf, garlic and salt in a the lard for five minutes, stirring often

- Add the sherry, wine and pepper and simmer until almost all the liquid has disappeared

- Add bone broth and simmer for 10 minutes

- Serve immediately or freeze for up to 6 months

## 2. Lemongrass and Carrot Soup

This is delicious served either hot or cold, and is especially satisfying during the winter.

### Ingredients

- 6 teaspoons lard or olive oil

- 1.5 cups onions, finely cut

- 24 oz. carrots, sliced

- 6 teaspoons fresh ground ginger

- 2 inch piece of lemongrass, crushed

- 1 liter Turkey Bone Broth

### Preparation Instructions

- Heat the lard in a saucepan and add the onions, cooking over medium heat for 8 minutes

- Introduce the ginger, carrots and crushed lemongrass and stir, cooking for 10 minutes

- Introduce the broth and simmer for 15 minutes

- Put the mixture in a food processor until it is smooth

- Add salt to taste and serve immediately or freeze for up to 6 months

# 3. Broiled Red Pepper Soup

This soup really brings out the Red Pepper's unique flavor, and serves well as both a side dish and a main meal.

## Ingredients

- 16 oz red bell peppers

- 3 teaspoons lard or olive oil

- 1 carrot, diced

- 1 leek, pale and white parts only, diced

- A diced celery stalk

- 1 teaspoon salt

- ½ teaspoon black pepper

- 6 teaspoons tomato puree

- 1.5 tablespoons sun-dried tomatoes

- 2 pints Turkey or Beef Bone Broth

- 1 cubed potato

## Preparation Method

- Broil the peppers on high heat for 8 minutes, turning them over until they are blackened on all sides

- Transfer them to a bowl and let them sit for 10 minutes

- Roughly chop the peppers

- Heat the oil or lard in a saucepan and introduce the peppers, carrot, leek, and celery for 10 minutes

- Add salt and black pepper to taste

- Add tomato puree and cook for 3 minutes, stirring often

- Introduce the thyme and tomatoes and heat for another 2 minutes

- Cover the mixture with the broth and potato, simmering for 20 minutes

- Use a food processor to smooth the mixture and serve immediately or store for six months

# 4. Chinese Style Sour Soup

This is just one variation of a very popular Asian style of soups. It works very well as a beverage as well as a starter to a meal.

## Ingredients

- 100 grams pork loin

- 0.25 cup dried lily flower

- 0.25 cup shiitake mushrooms

- 0.25 cup Bamboo Shoots

- 0.25 cup rice vinegar

- 0.25 cup arrowroot powder

- 0.5 teaspoon lard or olive oil

- 0.75 cup water

- 4 pints Pork or Turkey Bone Broth

- 0.25 teaspoon cayenne pepper

- 0.5 teaspoon white pepper

- 2 teaspoons soy sauce

- Salt

- 2 eggs, beaten

- 1 roughly cut scallion

## Preparation Method

- Cut the pork into small pieces

- Soak the flowers and mushrooms in water for 10 minutes then cut into small pieces

- Boil 7.25 cups of broth, add the pork and stir

- Introduce the peppers, soy sauce, salt, lily, mushrooms, shoots, sesame oil and vinegar

- In a different saucepan, heat the lard  and add arrowroot powder

- Using the remaining broth, make a slurry using the arrowroot powder mixture

- Slowly add the slurry to the main soup

- Introduce the eggs to the soup, stirring constantly

- Cook for 5 minutes and serve or freeze for up to 6 months

## 5. Rich Chicken soup

This recipe is a reminder that anything can evolve to provide you with new and exciting experiences. It comes in two parts, a broth, and the complete soup

**Ingredients**

*For the Broth*

- 1 tablespoon lard or olive oil

- 2 chicken breasts, skinless and boneless

- 2 chicken thighs, skinless and boneless

- 2 diced onions

- 2 bay leaves

- 1 small piece of turmeric, roughly chopped

- 3 roughly chopped garlic cloves

- 2 teaspoons salt

- 1.5 pints Chicken Bone Broth

*For the soup*

- 3 teaspoons lard or olive oil

- 3 sliced carrots

- 2 sliced celery stalks

- 1 teaspoon fresh thyme

- Salt to taste

## Preparation Method

*The Broth*

- Heat the lard in a large saucepan and fry the chicken until it is brown on both sides

- Add the onions and cook for 3 minutes

- Introduce the bay leaves, garlic, turmeric, salt, and half a pint of bone broth and simmer for 20 minutes

- Add the remaining bone broth and simmer for 15 minutes

- Remove the chicken breasts and simmer for another 10 minutes

- Strain the mixture and let it sit for 5 minutes

*The Soup*

- Clean the saucepan and heat the lard

- Cook the carrots and celery for 5 minutes

- Put in the thyme with 30 seconds left to go

- Add the broth and simmer for 5 minutes

- Serve immediately or freeze for up to 6 months

# 6. Spicy Tom Yum

Inspired by the tastes of Thailand, this Tom Yum recipe borrows from the original, but adds a few new flavors to create a unique experience.

## Ingredients

- 2 pints Chicken or Turkey Bone Broth

- 3 stalks of lemongrass, cut into 5 cm pieces

- One small piece of ginger, finely sliced

- 2 fresh red chilies

- 6 teaspoons fish Sauce

- 10 ml honey

- ½ lbs straw mushrooms

- 1 lbs jumbo shrimp

- Rind of 2 limes

- Juice from 2 limes

- 2 scallions, diced

- 6 teaspoons chopped cilantro

- Salt

## Preparation Method

- Put the broth, chilies, lemongrass and ginger in a large saucepan and simmer for 15 minutes, then remove the lemongrass and ginger

- Introduce the fish sauce, mushrooms and honey and simmer for 5 minutes

- Put in the shrimps and cook until they turn pink

- Remove from the heat and add the lime rind and juice, the scallions and the cilantro

- Add salt to taste and serve immediately or freeze for up to 6 months

# 7. Prawn Bisque

Bisque is a soup that uses ground or powdered crustacean shells. Though traditionally served with rice, this recipe utilizes squash as a way to avoid gluten.

## Ingredients

- 1 small squash, finely chopped

- 2 teaspoons salt

- 3 teaspoons lard or olive oil

- 1 finely chopped carrot

- 1 finely sliced leek

- 3 crushed garlic cloves

- 1 lb shelled prawns (keep the shells)

- 3 teaspoons tomato puree

- 2 fl oz brandy

- 4 fl oz sherry

- 0.25 teaspoon black pepper

- 1.5 pints Shrimp Stock

## Preparation Method

- In a large saucepan, combine the squash, stock and half the salt and simmer to soften the squash

- Place the mixture into a food processor and blend until smooth

- Using the same saucepan, heat the lard and add the carrot, leek, garlic and salt over medium heat for 5 minutes

- Introduce the prawn shells and tomato puree and cook for 5 minutes, stirring occasionally

- Include the cognac and sherry, and simmer for 5 minutes

- In another saucepan, put the shrimp stock, squash, black pepper and salt, and cook for 5 minutes

- Place the mixture in a food processor and blend until smooth

- Strain the blended mixture back into the saucepan

- Introduce the shrimp and cook for 5 minutes. Serve immediately

# 8. Lobster and Chorizo Stew

People see lobster as a "Rich Man's" food. This recipe is anything but, yet still manages to maintain the delicate flavor of the lobster.

## Ingredients

- 6 teaspoons lard or butter

- 1 shallot, minced

- 3 garlic cloves, crushed

- 2 teaspoons salt

- 4 branches thyme, leaves chopped

- 4 fl oz. vermouth

- 2 links chorizo, finely sliced

- 1 finely chopped sweet potato

- 0.5 teaspoon saffron

- 1.5 pints Chicken Bone Broth

- 2 lobster tails

## Preparation Method

- Heat the lard in a large saucepan and add the shallot, salt and garlic

- Cook over medium heat for 5 minutes, stirring intermittently

- Introduce thyme and vermouth, and wait for vermouth to evaporate

- Put in the chorizo, sweet potato, bone broth and saffron and simmer until the potato is soft

- Introduce the lobster tails and cook for 2 minutes

- Take out tails and remove their meat

- Chop the meat and put it back in the pot for 5 minutes

- Serve immediately

# 9. Coconut Chicken Stew with Lime and Ginger

This meal is great for summer, and is so easy to make it can be made in one pan.

## Ingredients

- 1 small onion, diced

- 3 teaspoons fresh crushed ginger

- 2 finely chopped garlic cloves

- 1 jalapeño pepper

- 1 13 oz can coconut milk

- 0.25 teaspoon honey

- 0.5 cup Cilantro

- 0.25 cup Chicken Bone Broth

- 6 teaspoons lard or ghee

- 3 lbs boneless chicken

- Salt

## Preparation Method

- Place the ginger, onion, garlic, pepper, coconut milk, honey, cilantro and broth in a food processor and smoothen, then set aside

- Season the chicken with salt

- Place the lard in a skillet and sear the chicken until golden brown

- Pour blended mixture into skillet and simmer for 20 minutes

- Serve immediately or store for up to 6 months

# 10. Curried Pork With Sweet Potatoes

This recipe is meant to help bring the curry out of the restaurant and into your kitchen.

## Ingredients

- 6 teaspoons lard

- 3 lbs pork cut into 3 inch cubes

- 2 teaspoons salt

- 9-12 teaspoons red curry paste

- 1 finely chopped onion

- Two 13 oz cans coconut milk

- 6 teaspoons fish sauce

- 5 finely chopped garlic cloves

- 1.5 pints Pork Bone Broth

- 2 finely chopped carrots

- 2 finely chopped sweet potatoes

- 2 tablespoons Cilantro

## Preparation Method

- Preheat oven to 350°F

- Heat the lard in an oven safe pot

- Season the pork with salt and sear until brown

- Put in curry paste, onion, coconut milk, fish sauce, garlic and broth and simmer for 5 minutes, then transfer to the oven for 2.5 hours

- Half an hour before it is ready, add the carrots and potatoes

- Leave the pot uncovered in the oven to thicken, and serve immediately.

# 11. Shellfish and Cactus Soup

The leaves from the Nopales, or Prickly Pear have numerous healing properties. Their antimicrobial, antioxidant, anti-inflammatory and neuroprotective properties make them some of the best-kept secrets your kitchen can ever have, and the benefit of adding them to bone broth is immense. The easiest place to get Nopales would be a Mexican market or an online store, though most supermarkets and health food stores will also sell them.

## Ingredients

- 2 pints Fish Bone Broth

- 4 average sized nopales

- 1 Chayote (a green squash, 8 tablespoons of peeled and diced celery or turnip can be used as a substitute)

- 2 white onions

- 2/3 tablespoon salt

- 4 guajillo peppers, dried (These are mild peppers but you could use fewer, or leave them out all together if you think they are too spicy)

- 2 cloves of garlic

- 3 teaspoons butter or lard

- 1 fl oz. olive oil

- 1 bunch cilantro, stemless

- 1.5 cups fresh bay scallops (frozen ones can also be used, but the fresher the better)

- 12 shrimp, halved

## Preparation Instructions

- Gently scrape away any of the prickly bits from the nopales paddles. Remember, they are very sharp so you need to exercise caution. Ensure that you cut any brown parts you see at the bottom of the stem.

- Wash each paddle thoroughly to ensure no more prickly thorns remain

- Cut the paddles into thin strips and wash them one more time (these three steps can be ignored if your local market or health food store sells the nopales precut)

- Remove the squash's outer cover and cut it into 1 inch cubes

- Wash the cubes in cold water

- Place the nopales and the squash in a medium sized saucepan and cover them with water

- Halve the onions, peel them, and place one half (whole) into the water with the nopales

- Add 1/3 tablespoon of salt

- Simmer the mixture for at least 20 minutes, then strain it. Do not mind the slightly viscous nature of the liquid, it is normal when cooking with cactus

- Remove the stems from the peppers and put them in a small saucepan.

- Submerge them in water and simmer for 10-15 minutes

- Strain the peppers and put them in a blender

- Add the garlic and ¾ pint of water to the blender

- Blend the mixture until smooth

- Cut the remaining onion (the half that you cut and the other one) into rings

- Melt the butter and 3 teaspoons olive oil in a stockpot

- Add the onion and stir fry until soft

- Add the cilantro and cook until the sprigs are flaccid

- Introduce the chayote, nopales and onion mix to the pot

- Add the last of the olive oil and stir

- Cover the mixture with the Fish Bone Broth and add the last of the salt

- Poor the blended peppers into the pot through a strainer

- Let the soup simmer for 10 – 15 minutes

- Add the scallops and shrimp and simmer until the shrimp are pink

- Serve immediately

To make this a truly Mexican dish, accompany the soup with some cubed avocado and tortilla chips. Add the fried chips to the soup so that they can soak it up to make it even more interesting. For those who think the  guajillo peppers do not pack enough of a punch, adding a few fresh jalapeños should do the trick.

# Chapter 4:
# Sauces

Bone broths can add richness to your sauces that will surprise you. In this chapter, we shall look at some of the bone-broth infused sauces that you can make at home.

## 1. Savory Ketchup

To get the best out of this recipe, it is important to use only the freshest tomatoes. If these are hard to get in your area, a can of San Marzano tomatoes should do.

### Ingredients

- 3 teaspoons olive oil

- 3 cups chopped carrots

- 1 diced yellow onion

- 5 teaspoons salt

- 1 teaspoon marjoram

- 0.25 teaspoon ground turmeric

- 1 teaspoon ground coriander

- 0.5 pint Turkey or Chicken Bone Broth

- 1 kg heirloom, San Marzano or Roma tomatoes

- 1 finely chopped red jalapeño

- 6 teaspoons white wine vinegar

- 3 teaspoons apple cider vinegar

**Preparation Method**

- Heat the olive oil in a saucepan, and put in the carrots, onion and 3 teaspoons of salt. Cook until browned, stirring intermittently

- Introduce the marjoram, turmeric, coriander and 1 teaspoon of salt and cook for 3 minutes, then simmer for 5 minutes

- Introduce the peppers, tomatoes, the last of the salt, and the vinegars and simmer for 20 minutes

- Blend the food in a food processor

- Strain the mixture and place back on the heat, simmering for 20 minutes.

- Let it cool to room temperature

- Store it in the fridge for 2 weeks, or in the freezer for a year

# 2. Tomato Jam

Many people do not realize that as a tomato can also be classified as a berry, you can also make jam with it. This recipe is just one way to do so.

## Ingredients

- 7 teaspoons salt

- 1 lb heirloom tomatoes

- 0.5 cup Chicken. Beef or Pork Bone Broth

- 6 teaspoons honey

- Squirt of fresh lemon juice

## Preparation Instructions

- Bring 2 pints of water to the boil and add 6 teaspoons of salt, and get a bowl of Ice water

- Remove the stalks of each tomato and slice an "X" at the base of every one

- Place the tomatoes in the hot water for 3 minutes, then transfer them to the ice bath to cool for the same amount of time

- Remove the skins and cut them into quarters

- Put them back into the saucepan and add honey, bone broth, lemon juice and the last teaspoon of salt

- Simmer for 25 minutes, stirring often

- Place the jam in storage containers and put them in the fridge for up to 2 weeks.

# 3. Beefy Barbecue Sauce

Barbecue sauce is often thought of as ketchup's cousin, and in this case, it may just be true.

## Ingredients

- 3 teaspoons lard

- 1 diced onion

- 1 crushed garlic clove

- 0.5 pint Savory Ketchup (see recipe above)

- 0.25 cup apple cider vinegar

- 0.25 cup honey

- 3 teaspoons molasses or maple syrup

- 0.25 teaspoon ground ginger

- 0.25 teaspoon dry mustard

- 0.5 teaspoon lime juice

- 2 teaspoons Worcestershire sauce

- 2 teaspoons tomato puree

- 0.25 cup Beef Bone Broth

## Preparation Method

- Heat the lard in a large pot and add the onion and garlic. Cook until semi-transparent

- Add bone broth and simmer for 5 minutes

- Introduce the rest of the ingredients, simmer for 10-15 minutes, until the sauce thickens

- Mix in a food processor until smooth

- Refrigerate for two weeks or freeze for a year

# 4. Zesty Barbecue Sauce

This sauce is inspired by Memphis style BBQ sauce, and is sure to become an instant hit.

## Ingredients

- 1 finely chopped onion

- 3 garlic cloves

- 3 teaspoons lard or coconut oil

- 0.5 pint Savory Ketchup (see recipe above)

- 3 teaspoons chili pepper

- 0.5 cup Pork Bone Broth

- 6 teaspoons Worcestershire sauce

- 6 teaspoons brewed coffee

- 6 teaspoons honey

- 3 teaspoons apple cider vinegar

- 1 lime rind

- Juice from one lime

## Preparation Method

- Place the lard in a saucepan and add the garlic and onions. Cook for 4 minutes

- Put in Ketchup and chilies and cook for 5 minutes

- Introduce the remaining ingredients and simmer for half an hour

- Put the mixture in a blender for 5 minutes

- Cool and refrigerate for 2 weeks or freeze for a year

# 5. Broth Infused Hot Sauce

Hot sauce has always helped to spice up a meal, and this recipe is no different.

## Ingredients

- 2 teaspoons lard or ghee

- 0.5 onion, diced

- 2 red chilies, diced

- 8 jalapeños, sliced

- 5 teaspoons crushed garlic

- 0.5 teaspoon salt

- 1 pint Chicken Bone Broth

- 8 fl oz. white vinegar

## Preparation Method

- Heat the lard in a large pot and add the onions. Cook until they are semi-transparent

- Add the chilies, jalapeños, garlic and salt and cook for five minutes

- Introduce the broth and simmer for 20 minutes

- Mix the result in a food processor, slowly adding the vinegar as you do so

- Cool the mixture and store it for later use. It will keep for 2 weeks in the refrigerator, and 1 year in the freezer

# 6. Beefy Red Wine Sauce

Red wine sauce goes well with any red meat, and this recipe adds a twist will leave your mouth watering.

## Ingredients

- 3 teaspoons lard or olive oil

- 0.25 cup shallot

- 4 fl oz red wine

- 4 fl oz port wine

- 4 fl oz Beef Bone Broth

- 3 teaspoons fresh rosemary

- Salt and pepper to taste

## Preparation Method

- Heat the lard in a large pot and add the shallots, cooking them for 3 minutes.

- Introduce the red and port wines and simmer until the liquid has dropped to ¾ its original volume

- Introduce the broth and simmer until liquid has gone down by ½

- Take it off the heat and serve immediately

# 7. Almond Infused Satay Sauce

Satay sauce is popular throughout the world, and this unique recipe substitutes the traditional peanut base with almond butter.

## Ingredients

- 0.5 cup finely sliced onion

- 3 teaspoons crushed garlic

- 3 teaspoons crushed ginger

- Pinch of pepper flakes

- 2 teaspoons lard or olive oil

- 2 teaspoons sesame oil

- 2 fl oz. Beef or Pork Bone Broth

- 3 teaspoons red wine vinegar

- 6 teaspoons honey

- 3 teaspoons soy sauce

- 0.25 cup almond butter

- 6 teaspoons Savory Ketchup

- 3 teaspoons dry sherry

- Grated rind from one lime

- Juice from one lime

**Preparation Method**

- Heat the lard in a large pot and mix the ginger, garlic, pepper flakes, onion, and sesame oil. Cook for 6 minutes

- Introduce the bone broth and begin to simmer

- Once simmering, introduce the remaining ingredients and wait 5 minutes for the mixture to thicken

- Blend the sauce until smooth and store in the refrigerator or freezer

# 8. Zesty Mango Chutney

Chutneys are condiments that originated in South Asia but are now popular throughout the world.

## Ingredients

- 0.75 teaspoon red pepper flakes

- 5 teaspoons lard or olive oil

- 1.5 finely sliced red onions

- 1 kg diced mangoes

- 0.25 cup fresh ground ginger

- 1 small diced red capsicum

- 0.5 teaspoon salt

- 4 fl oz Beef or Pork bone broth

- 4 fl oz. unsweetened pineapple juice

- 2 fl oz. apple cider vinegar

- 0.25 cup honey

- 2 teaspoons curry powder

- Ground black pepper to taste

- 0.25 cup raisins

- 0.25 cup currants

## Preparation Method

- Toast the pepper flakes in a pan for 5 minutes

- Introduce the lard, onions, mangoes, ginger, capsicum, and salt and cook for 5 minutes

- Slowly introduce the broth, pineapple juice, apple cider vinegar, honey, curry powder and black pepper, stirring occasionally

- Introduce the currants and raisins, and simmer for half an hour

- Serve immediately or store for up to 2 weeks in the refrigerator

# 9. Bacon Relish

Almost everyone loves bacon, and those who do not like it have probably not tasted it yet. This recipe is therefore sure to be a hit among friends and family

## Ingredients

- 4 strips of bacon

- 1 finely sliced onion

- 2 fl oz. Beef bone broth

- 3 cloves garlic, crushed

- 0.25 cup raisins

## Preparation Method

- Pan fry the bacon to get it crispy, and drain on paper towels

- Using 3 teaspoons of bacon fat, fry the onion for 10 minutes or until caramelized

- Introduce the broth and simmer for 4 minutes

- Introduce the garlic and raisins and simmer for a minute

- Puree the mixture in a food processor, then add the bacon and blend until the bacon is roughly cut

- Serve immediately on burgers or hotdogs, or store in the refrigerator for up to 1 week.

# 10. Red Salsa

This is the perfect hot sauce for the table, mild yet flavorful, with an earthy tone that complements beef especially well,

## Ingredients

- A Puya chili

- 0.25 onion, finely chopped

- 0.5 jalapeño

- 1 garlic clove

- 8 fl oz bone broth (any flavor will do)

- 8 fl oz. Savory Ketchup

- 4 sprigs cilantro cut fine

- Salt to taste

- 1 pint water

## Preparation Method

- Bring the water to the boil and introduce the Puya chili. Take off the heat and let it stand for 10 minutes

- Take out the chili and throw away the water

- Mix chili with the remaining ingredients in a blender and mix until smooth

- Place the mixture in a saucepan and simmer for 20 minutes

- Serve immediately or store in an airtight container in the refrigerator for up to two weeks.

# Conclusion

If you begin to use the recipes in this book, you will begin to understand why Bone Broths have become so popular over such a short amount of time. The trend is not going to go anywhere anytime soon, as the possibilities are endless, and the benefits are still being discovered.

Despite the skepticism surrounding the Bone Broth movement, the popularity of bone broth is on the rise, and more people are beginning to understand how they can integrate it into their normal diet. I hope that the recipes in this book will help you see why being health conscious does not always have to be boring.